How to Start Running
(And Enjoy It)

How to Start Running (And Enjoy It)

Three-Month Run-Walk
Training Program for Everyone

Sarah Austin Casson

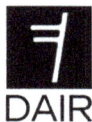

DAIR

Library of Congress Control Number: 2024900619

This publication is designed to provide running guidance but not medical advice. Readers should consult with a medical professional before starting this training program. Mention of specific companies, organizations, or authorities in this book does not imply endorsement by the author or publisher, nor does mention of specific companies, organizations, or authorities imply that they endorse this book, its author, or the publisher.

Internet addresses given in this book were accurate at the time it went to press.

Book Design by Sarah Lahay

First Edition 2024
ISBN: 9798218307059 (ebook)
ISBN: 9798218307042 (paperback)

Published by Dair Press
Berkeley, California
www.DairPress.com

Dair Press
A publishing company founded on intellectual curiosity and a sense of adventure.

For Fiona

Hello Friend!

So, you want to start running? That is great! Running can bring you all sorts of accomplishments, adventures, new friends, and physical and emotional health—and I promise that it can be fun. You'll start to see some benefits almost right away, and all of them will keep adding up over time. Take it from me: I've been running for more than twenty years and have helped countless others become runners themselves! We run because it's fun and rewarding. Follow this training plan and you'll find yourself having an enjoyable time running too.

Usually when someone gets into running they do too much too soon: They run a mile super fast, and it is painful, miserable, and much slower than they thought they could run. They get discouraged and incredibly sore. That's no fun. I have a better way! Start slowly and be consistent. It will feel like nothing at first, and then before you know it, you will be running multiple times a week like it is no big deal. And the best part? It will be enjoyable. By the end of these three months, you will actually be looking forward to your runs.

You've Got This!

My three-month, run-walk program will take you from walking for thirty minutes to comfortably running for thirty minutes three times a week.

Throughout the three months, each workout should feel easy, probably almost too easy—and that's good! The program helps you slowly trick yourself into running more and more, allowing your body plenty of time to adjust and adapt.

When you complete the program, I've got a few suggestions at the end of this book for what running training you could do next.

Hot Tip: Accountability Buddies
Make running even more fun by doing it
with friends, in person or remotely. And by
friends I mean an accountability buddy—
or three. Accountability buddies can run
together and get coffee afterward.
If your accountability buddies are remote,
I highly recommend a text chain solely
devoted to photos of yourself or your
surroundings post-run.
The key is to keep the running fun—
and friends help make things fun!

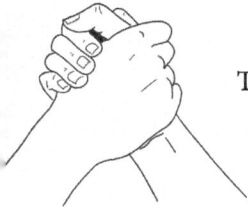

Before You Start

Before you begin this program, it is important that you can walk for thirty minutes at a time, relatively comfortably, three times a week. If that is not where you are at right now, it's all good. Begin by gently building up your walking duration and chat with your doctor about how best to do that. Then once you are there, come back and start this training program.

What's Included in This Book

- A list of the gear you will want and where to get it
- Important running tips and tricks
- Optional reflection pages to record where you are when you start your training
- A running program for the next three months
- Weekly training log pages
- Optional reflection pages to track where you are at the end of the three months

What You Need

- Running bra (if you wear one)
- Running shoes
- Running clothes
- A timer (This can be a watch or a phone.)

Just Thirty Minutes at a Time

This training plan has you alternating walking and running for thirty minutes at a time, three times a week. During those thirty minutes you will do five repetitions of running and walking. Every two weeks you will increase the amount you run and decrease the amount you walk. By week 11 of the plan, you'll be running for thirty minutes straight, without needing to walk.

Example

Week 1: You walk for 5 minutes, then run for 1 minute. You repeat this for 5 repetitions, a total of thirty minutes. The shorthand for such a workout is written in this training program as **5w/1r x 5**.

At the start of Week 3: You bump up to 4 minutes of walking and 2 minutes of running. You repeat this for 5 repetitions, a total of thirty minutes. The shorthand is **4w/2r x 5**.

Cross-Training

Twice a week you will be doing additional non-running workouts (cross-training). You get to pick what this is. More on this can be found in the Important Running Tips and Tricks section of this book.

Tracking Your Runs and Workouts

It can be helpful to track what you do each day throughout this program. In the weekly log, I've included what you are supposed to do each day that week and space for you to write down what runs and cross-training workouts you actually did. Take the time to write these things down. It can be a pain, but it will be helpful to see what you did each day and week—and understand your trends over time. Writing down what you accomplished each day of the training program also makes it more likely that you'll stick to the prescribed schedule.

In the weekly log, I have also included room for you to write notes on your cross-training workouts, your sleep, your mental health, and any aches or potential injuries. Sleep and mental health are important for your life in general, and they both help—and are helped by—running. If you like writing notes about these running-adjacent things, great. If not, just ignore those sections of the weekly training log.

Again, I Promise You've Got This!

Follow this training plan and pretty soon you'll find yourself running for an entire thirty minutes at a time—and having fun while you're at it. I believe in you!

Happy Running!
Sarah

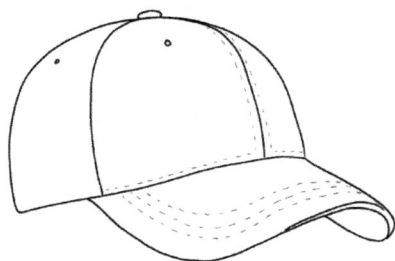

Gear You Will Want and Where to Find It

I've been running for more than twenty years, so I've tried all the different things and made many silly mistakes. I've run in suburban neighborhoods, in dense cities, in high mountain peaks, in the desert, in very cold, snowy winters, on tropical islands, and in jungles around the world. I've tried lots of gear in lots of places. Below are my recommendations of what I think you'll need and want for this training plan, regardless of where you're located. I'm not sponsored—I just like products from good brands, many of which you'll see mentioned below.

Hat

Any hat that you like wearing is perfect. I have seven-year-old hat that is disgusting with sweat, and it is the most comfortable thing ever. I love it.

Sunglasses

Eye protection is important, especially if it is sunny. Any pair of sunglasses that you like will do just great. I run in my prescription sunglasses that are supposed to be children's cycling sunglasses. (I have a small head!) You might like your beat-up beach sunglasses or a wearing a run-specific brand that comes with fancy features, like wraparound frames, interchangeable lenses, and a lightweight feel. Some good brands to consider are Goodr, Roka, Nathan, and Oakleys.

Beyond UV protection for your eyes, what matters the most is that the sunglasses fit on your face. You want to be sure they won't fall off with sweat and don't start hurting your ears twenty minutes into a run. What works great for your friend or a random person on the internet might not work for you— or maybe it does! If possible, try on sunglasses in person at a running shop, an outdoor gear store, or an optometrist office.

Clothing

Running-specific shirts, shorts and socks will likely make your run more comfortable. Winter running and summer running clothing can differ greatly. You can run in whatever you want. Jorts? Sure. You might already have a perfectly good t-shirt in your closet already. You can get quite fancy with running clothes. If you want to do that, great. If you don't, no need.

The only time running clothing matters a lot is when the weather is extremely hot or extremely cold. But, uh, that also might not be fun weather to start running in. So set yourself up for success: It's a lot easier to start running in nice weather than to have to figure out how to deal with extreme weather and start running.

But that's not always possible. You might live some-where with extreme weather and have to adjust your runs (and outfits) to the elements. Or maybe it is January 1st and you just want get started, regardless of the snow flurries. If that's your case, make sure to do a bit of research first about your specific weather-related clothing needs. All of the clothing and shoe companies mentioned in this Gear section will be more than happy to point you in the right direction. Online magazines, like Trail Runner and Runner's World, will have good articles on how to dress for every different type of weather condition. With the right gear, (almost) all weather is enjoyable to run in! Some weather just requires a bit more prep.

A reminder: If it's a blizzard or really hot outside, a treadmill is always a good option—and can be used for every single run of this plan.

For all your running clothing needs, some good companies to check out: Oiselle, Outdoor Voices, Patagonia, Lululemon, Nathan, Craft, and Brooks. Explore what is stocked in your local REI and running stores.

Running Shorts or Tights

Shorts will work just fine in most weather. If it is very cold, wear some yoga leggings or fancy cold-weather-specific running tights. If you don't already own some you love, Oiselle or REI is probably your best bet here. Be on the lookout for sales.

I prefer lightweight shorts. I tend to alternate between my (both very old) bright orange Craft shorts and my hot pink Outdoor Voices ones. Questions to consider before venturing into purchasing running-specific shorts: Do you want to carry things in your shorts? Are you looking for modesty coverage? Do you prefer that almost-nothing feel while moving around? Do exercise shorts tend to chafe your inner thighs?

Outdoor Voices makes shorts with a back pocket that is great for carrying a phone. Oiselle makes great longer-length shorts and almost all of their shorts come with pockets. Any running shorts termed "fly away" will give you that almost-nothing feel; Lululemon makes them, as does Nathan, Craft, and a lot more. If you get chafing, consider running in compression shorts, like Lululemon's Align, Outdoor Voices' Warmup or Oiselle's Wyomia—all of these will have minimal seams and are made not to move around that much against your legs.

Running Shirts

If you don't already own running shirts that you love, Oiselle has some great ones. Buy them online or at REI. For both hot and cold weather, I prefer wool shirts. They take A LOT longer to stink up than do synthetic or cotton shirts, tend to hold up longer over the years, and wick sweat/dry much faster than other materials.

> For warmer weather: a lightweight, breathable shirt will make you more comfortable.

For colder weather: **throw a sweatshirt on over your shirt.**

If it is extremely cold, get a breathable jacket designed specifically for running. Depending on where you are, it should be windproof and/or waterproof. Oiselle and REI both sell great options.

Watch/Phone

You will want to keep track of your intervals of running/walking for a given run. Use a watch or a phone for this.

You don't need a fancy watch, but if you want one, get one. I use a Garmin, but I also love the Timex ones that have simple timers. You can find one for less than fifty dollars.

Or use your phone to track the time with an interval app. The iPhone app "Simple Interval Timer" is free and can be programmed to keep you on track for each run and walk section of the workout's thirty minutes. Android has similar apps.

I have recommendations on how to run with a phone in the next section, Important Running Tips and Tricks!

Sunscreen

If you live in an super sunny place, figuring out what sunscreen you like to use for running is important. If you don't already have a go-to, try different ones out. A few brands to start with are Coppertone, Neutrogena, Hawaiian Sol, and ThinkSport.

You can also get shirts with a high UPF rating (similar to the SPF ratings of sunscreen). They are made from a breathable fabric that is woven in a way to protect you from the sun. Oiselle, Patagonia, and many other companies make this type of shirt.

Bras

If you're a bra-wearing human, get yourself a running-specific bra. A good bra makes a world of difference. Bouncing boobs make for an unfun run. Luckily, this industry has exploded in the last couple of years, and there are now a ton of options out there for every body and boob.

Most running stores and REI will have a large selection of different bras to try on. Look for ones labeled "high impact." I'd suggest considering Knix's Catalyst bra for size D or larger. Try several styles in the size bra you normally wear. Jump up and down a lot and see how each one feels to you. If it doesn't feel good as you jump around in the store, it won't feel good on a run.

Online purchasing is also a great option. Some good places to start are Oiselle, Brooks, Outdoor Voices, and REI. My favorite for running bras is Outdoor Voices.

The company, Koala Clip, makes a Sports Bra Phone Pouch that'll let you easily tuck your phone, credit card, keys, whatever into the back of your bra. Not a necessity but can be a nice extra when you don't have pockets.

Socks

I think wool socks are the best. Yes, even in the summer. Wool wicks sweat away, so your feet will stay dry even as you sweat. Dry feet mean less chance of getting blisters. You can find good thick ones for winter and thin ones for summer. Try some different styles to see what you like best. Consider sock height, material, and compression. My favorite pair: Patagonia's Wool Anklet Socks.

Socks can be surprisingly expensive, but they make a world of a difference. Comfortable feet make for a much better run. That said, like all these recommendations, whatever feels best to you is your best bet. That might be what you already own and wear as socks in everyday life.

Shoes

Running shoes are SUPER IMPORTANT. Don't just buy any pair of sneakers or run in your old Converses from the closet. Go purchase shoes specifically for running. Every major city has multiple stores dedicated to the sole practice of selling shoes for running. Visit one.

Expect to spend thirty to sixty minutes trying on shoes during your first visit to a running shoe store. An employee will likely ask you to run on their treadmill to test out the shoes and watch how your feet hit the ground with each step.

In-store assessments provide good information, but the most important test is which pair feel the best on your feet as you walk around. Nothing else matters as much as that does. There's a lot of jargon involved in selling running shoes (e.g., weight, stability, cushion, motion control, etc.). That matters only a tiny bit compared to how you feel when moving around in the shoes.

Get new running shoes every 300 to 500 miles. I promise if you keep running, you will hit that mileage and can feel extra proud of yourself as you go buy your second pair!

Hot Tip: Orthotics

If you need orthotics, don't buy them in a running store. Generic, out-of-the-box orthotics are nonsense—even the ones that promise to be customized to your feet by being heated in-store. If you need orthotics, go to a podiatrist and get some made explicitly for your needs.

My favorite orthotics are Sole Supports. They are a million times better than all the other orthotics (and I have tried a lot). Find a podiatrist who makes Sole Supports orthotics by going to their website (SoleSupports.com).

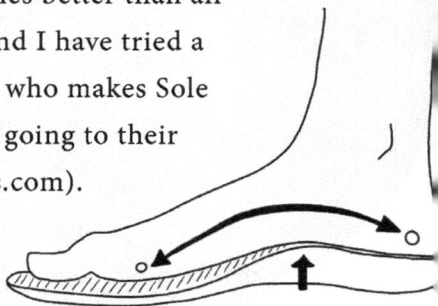

Running Backpack or Belt

Try to carry as little as possible during a run, while still feeling comfortable and safe.

A backpack or belt is not necessary for this training plan, but they can be nice, especially if you are taking the subway back and forth to where you want to run. I don't like running with things in my pockets, so I have a small running belt (a.k.a. a fanny pack) for runs under forty-five minutes. I use a running backpack with a water bladder for longer runs. Both basically just hold things for me.

A running pack or belt is a subjective choice and depends on your preference. If you are not sure, just go for your run and see: If you wish you had brought more stuff with you or find that you don't like your subway metro card shoved in your pocket with your keys, running with a belt or backpack may be the answer. And, if you are wondering if you should get a running belt or a backpack . . . get a running belt.

Check out the supply of running packs and belts at REI. If you go in person or call them on the phone, they can steer you to an option that works well for you. And, they have a good return policy, so if your first choice is uncomfortable you can always return it and try another one. A regular fanny pack (or backpack) also works. Sometimes they get a bit bouncy and flop about, which can be annoying and is why people buy running-specific ones.

Reflective Clothing and Lights for Dawn, Dusk, and Nighttime Running

If you plan on running at dawn, dusk, or night, please wear reflective clothing and a light (or two). Do not assume that cars can see you. The little strip of reflective tape that comes on most running shoes does not make your visible to drivers. Just a headlamp is not enough for a car to see you, especially from behind.

REI and Oiselle both have a great selection of reflective clothing, gear, and lights to make you visible to others.

You'll also want some extra lighting for your own eyes. Wearing a headlamp or a attaching a clip-on flashlight to your shorts will help light up your running path, making it less likely that you'll trip over some uneven sidewalk or a stray branch.

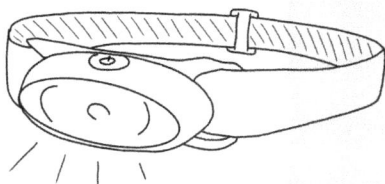

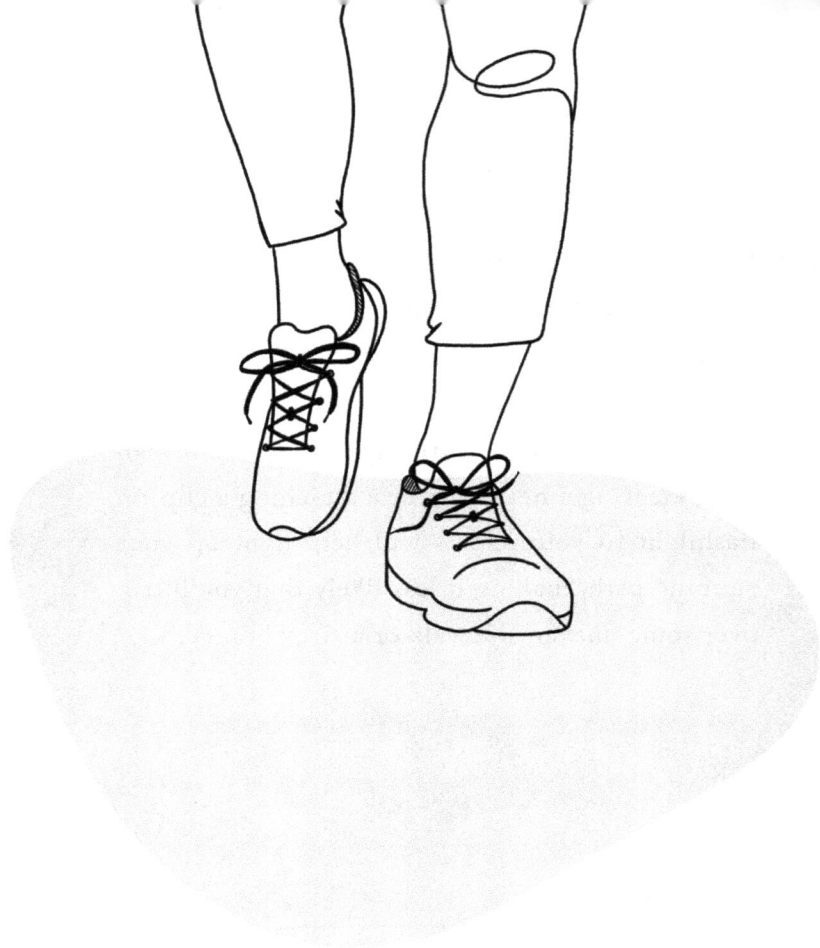

Important Running Tips and Tricks

Hydration

You don't need to carry water with you on the runs for this training program. It is important to pay attention to your hydration though. If you are running somewhere really remote and might get lost for a day or two, or if you are running somewhere very dry (like the desert), or if your run is more than fifteen miles (again, not this training program), then it is a good idea to have water with you.

If you are not in one of those three scenarios but still getting thirsty on your runs, that is a sign you are not drinking enough water throughout the day.

Managing Dehydration

Common signs of dehydration are dark yellow pee, not peeing that much, feeling dizzy, dry mouth, and headache. Preventing dehydration can be as easy as getting into the habit of bringing a water bottle around with you. Sip on it often throughout the day.

If you are dehydrated, you need to replenish your water levels *and* your electrolytes. Drink water as well as sports drinks, such as Gatorade. You can also drink rehydration salts mixed into water. Companies like Nuun, GU, and Liquid I.V. make decent-enough tasting rehydration salt powers and tablets to easily add to a glass of water. My favorite way to hydrate: throw a few dashes of salt, a squeeze of lemon juice, and some grated ginger into coconut water.

When recovering from dehydration, be sure to rehydrate steadily for a few days. You should start feeling better pretty quickly. If you don't start feeling better within a few hours, seek medical attention. Unchecked dehydration will kill you, but the chances of that happening are quite low. Just drink some fluids, chat with a doctor if necessary, and you will be fine.

Hot Tip: Drink Up!
Becoming dehydrated means that something is not right in what you are doing on a regular basis. Likely, you are not consuming enough water throughout the day or did not get enough electrolytes to balance how much you sweated them out. Be especially **careful about** this on **super hot days.**

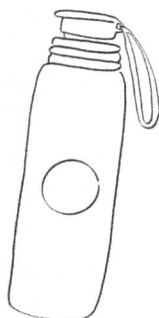

Nutrition

Eat whatever works for your body now. The general rules of nutrition apply to running: Get your body some fruits, veggies, protein, fiber, and healthy fats. However you do that is great.

Personally, my stomach cannot handle digesting anything within an hour before I run, and I get really nauseous if I push it. Your stomach may be different from mine. As you continue running, you will figure out what works for you regarding food intake and running. If you like tracking data or journaling, recording what food you eat and when, can help you identify trends over time. (Was the banana thirty minutes before the run fine but the oatmeal wasn't?)

After you finish a run, you want to eat some form of a complex carbohydrate, protein and good fat within thirty minutes. (My favorite is a tasty smoothie.) Those thirty minutes are a special window to replenish your glycogen levels, which translates to better and easier recovery from your run. That said, more important than that thirty minute post-run window is eating good nutrition throughout the day.

Stretching

Stretch after every run, ideally for fifteen to thirty minutes. There are countless types of stretching, so take some time to figure out what works for you. Start by Googling: "How to stretch for running." Try out various approaches and see what feels best to your body. Start with focusing on your quads, butt, and hips.

Yoga is also a good way to learn proper stretching techniques. YouTube has lots of follow-along videos, and in-person classes are always great. Having a teacher correct your form can help a lot.

Foam Rolling

Coupling your stretching (and maybe yoga) with some foam rolling is not necessary, but some people really like it. It can help tight IT bands, hamstrings, quads, and calves. You can buy a foam roller at REI or many other places online. Learn how to self-massage your muscles from the instructions that come with the foam roller—and check YouTube for lots of instructional videos.

Run Slower Than You Think You Should

How fast should you be running these runs? The simple answer is: Run slower than you think you should. Don't sprint. Take it at a casual, slower-than-you-expect pace.

Aim for a slow jog where you could chat the entire time. You will have a lot more fun this way, and science promises that by keeping your pace slow, you will actually get faster over time at the same effort level.

Eventually, if you keep running over the years, you will want to add in some faster-paced runs, such as a sprint workout. But those harder runs should happen at most only once or twice a week. Serious runners and even top professionals, who run six days a week, only do one or two fast workouts per week. Most of their runs are super gentle—and you should treat yourself the same way. Do not run hard or fast for any of the workouts in this training program.

For this training program, if you are absolutely exhausted next day after running, you went too hard or fast. Take it easier next time. Being gentle on yourself will make it more fun.

Phone

Some people run with a phone. Some don't. I don't run with my phone very often, but there are plenty of good reasons to bring it with you: safety, getting lost, tracking your route, tracking your run/walk timing, calling a Lyft, listening to music/audiobook/ podcast, etc.

If you run with your phone, be thoughtful about where you place it on your body. It looks light, but if you carry on the wrong part of your body, you will mess up how you swing your arms and legs as you run. This increases your chance of injuring yourself. Keep your phone positioned as close to the center of your lower torso as possible.

Hot Tip: Running with a Phone

If you are running with your phone, keep it close to the center of your torso. Ideally, place it on your lower torso unless you're stashing it in your bra with something like the Koala Clip.

DON'T

- Carry your phone in your hand. Even something as light as keys in your hands will throw off your running alignment.
- Wear it in an armband.
- Carry it in the side pocket on your shorts or leggings.

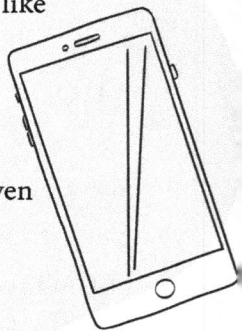

DO
- Carry your phone in a fanny pack or running belt.
- Wear it in your short's lower back pocket that is specifically made to carry a phone ergonomically on a run.
- Clip it to the back of your bra with something like the Koala Clip.
- Consider leaving it at home.

Headphones

If you run with headphones make sure you can still hear traffic and be extra aware of your surroundings.

Running with only one earbud in seems safer but is actually worse. Your brain does not process the two forms of noise (the traffic and whatever you're listening to) as clearly as it would with both earbuds in. Running with only one earbud in makes you less likely to hear that car coming.

I don't run with headphones, but plenty of people enjoy listening to something as they run. You do you.

Cross-Training

You will see in your weekly training log that there are two cross-training workouts each week. These can be any physical activity you want and should range from thirty to sixty minutes.

Go rock climbing or surfing. Take a walk in the park or a yoga class. Try lifting upper body weights and adding more stretching to your routine (beyond the stretching you do after a run). Kinda anything that gets your body moving counts.

When choosing your cross-training activity, pay attention to how your body is feeling: choose a gentle workout if you need some recovery or do something more rigorous if your body is up for it.

I Could Not Get to a Run This Week! What Should I Do?

Not a big deal. Just repeat that week's schedule for the following week—thus extending the program to 13 weeks. Moving onto the next week's program after skipping workouts will increase your chances of getting injured. No need for that!

Okay So I Am Running, Does This Mean I Have to Sign Up for a Race?

Nope. One of the most beautiful parts of running is the utter purposeless purpose to it. The only point to running is your health and enjoyment. If that includes goals like races, great. If not, don't even worry about it.

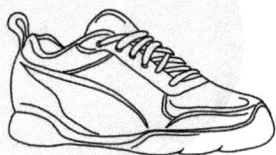

Reflections
Before You Start the Three-Month Training Program

Why am I doing this?

What am I excited about?

Is there anything that am I nervous about?

What do I expect to learn from these three months?

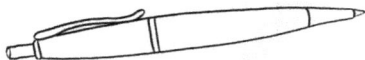

3-Month Training Program Overview

Every running workout in this plan is thirty minutes, for a total of ninety minutes of running per week.

> Remember: **Don't sprint the runs.**
> Take it even easier than you think you
> should. Slower is better here.

Cross-training activity and lengths are up to you. Listen to your body to determine the best intensity for you.

5w/1r x5 = Walk for 5 minutes, run for 1 minute. Repeat that 5 times, so spend thirty minutes in total.

	Day 1	Day 2	Day 3
Week 1	5w/1r x5	*Cross-Training*	5w/1r x5
Week 2	*Cross-Training*	5w/1r x5	*Cross-Training*
Week 3	4w/2r x5	*Cross-Training*	4w/2r x5
Week 4	*Cross-Training*	4w/2r x5	*Cross-Training*
Week 5	3w/3r x5	*Cross-Training*	3w/3r x5
Week 6	*Cross-Training*	3w/3r x5	*Cross-Training*
Week 7	2w/4r x5	*Cross-Training*	2w/4r x5
Week 8	*Cross-Training*	2w/4r x5	*Cross-Training*
Week 9	1w/5r x5	*Cross-Training*	1w/5r x5
Week 10	*Cross-Training*	1w/5r x5	*Cross-Training*
Week 11	Run 30 Minutes	*Cross-Training*	Run 30 Minutes
Week 12	*Cross-Training*	Run 30 Minutes	*Cross-Training*

Day 4	Day 5	Day 6	Day 7
Cross-Training	REST	5w/1r x5	REST
5w/1r x5	REST	5w/1r x5	REST
Cross-Training	REST	4w/2r x5	REST
4w/2r x5	REST	4w/2r x5	REST
Cross-Training	REST	3w/3r x5	REST
3w/3r x5	REST	3w/3r x5	REST
Cross-Training	REST	2w/4r x5	REST
2w/4r x5	REST	2w/4r x5	REST
Cross-Training	REST	1w/5r x5	REST
1w/5r x5	REST	1w/5r x5	REST
Cross-Training	REST	Run 30 Minutes	REST
Run 3 Miles*	REST	Run 30 Minutes	REST

Yes, this one is different! It lets you see what it feels like to run by miles, not minutes. You might prefer one over the other. And you might surprise yourself that three miles is not actually as far as you might have thought it was eleven weeks ago!

Weekly
Training
Log

Week 1

What Was Scheduled	What You Actually Did
DAY 1: **5w/1r x 5** (Walk for 5 minutes, run for 1 minute. Repeat that 5 times, so spend thirty minutes in total.)	
DAY 2: **Cross-Training**	
DAY 3: **5w/1r x 5**	
DAY 4: **Cross-Training**	
DAY 5: **Rest**	
DAY 6: **5w/1r x 5**	
DAY 7: **Rest**	

How did this week's runs go? Did I like them?
How did they make me feel?

What did I do for each cross-training workout?
Did I like it? How did it make me feel?

How much sleep did I get this week?
Was it enough?

How was my mental health this week?

Does anything hurt or feel sore on my body? If so, what have I done about it? (e.g., stretch, massage, etc.)

Anything else?

Week 2

What Was Scheduled	What You Actually Did
DAY 1: Cross-Training	
DAY 2: 5w/1r x 5	
DAY 3: Cross-Training	
DAY 4: 5w/1r x 5	
DAY 5: Rest	
DAY 6: 5w/1r x 5	
DAY 7: Rest	

How did this week's runs go? Did I like them?
How did they make me feel?

What did I do for each cross-training workout?
Did I like it? How did it make me feel?

How much sleep did I get this week?

Was it enough?

How was my mental health this week?

Does anything hurt or feel sore on my body? If so, what have I done about it? (e.g., stretch, massage, etc.)

Anything else?

Week 3

What Was Scheduled	What You Actually Did
DAY 1: 4w/2r x 5	
DAY 2: Cross-Training	
DAY 3: 4w/2r x 5	
DAY 4: Cross-Training	
DAY 5: Rest	
DAY 6: 4w/2r x 5	
DAY 7: Rest	

How did this week's runs go? Did I like them?
How did they make me feel?

What did I do for each cross-training workout?
Did I like it? How did it make me feel?

How much sleep did I get this week?
Was it enough?

How was my mental health this week?

Does anything hurt or feel sore on my body? If so,
what have I done about it? (e.g., stretch, massage, etc.)

Anything else?

Week 4

What Was Scheduled	What You Actually Did
DAY 1: Cross-Training	
DAY 2: 4w/2r x 5	
DAY 3: Cross-Training	
DAY 4: 4w/2r x 5	
DAY 5: Rest	
DAY 6: 4w/2r x 5	
DAY 7: Rest	

How did this week's runs go? Did I like them?
How did they make me feel?

What did I do for each cross-training workout?
Did I like it? How did it make me feel?

How much sleep did I get this week?
Was it enough?

How was my mental health this week?

Does anything hurt or feel sore on my body? If so, what have I done about it? (e.g., stretch, massage, etc.)

Anything else?

Week 5

What Was Scheduled	What You Actually Did
DAY 1: 3w/3r x 5	
DAY 2: Cross-Training	
DAY 3: 3w/3r x 5	
DAY 4: Cross-Training	
DAY 5: Rest	
DAY 6: 3w/3r x 5	
DAY 7: Rest	

How did this week's runs go? Did I like them?
How did they make me feel?

What did I do for each cross-training workout?
Did I like it? How did it make me feel?

How much sleep did I get this week?
Was it enough?

How was my mental health this week?

Does anything hurt or feel sore on my body? If so, what have I done about it? (e.g., stretch, massage, etc.)

Anything else?

Week 6

What Was Scheduled	What You Actually Did
DAY 1: Cross-Training	
DAY 2: 3w/3r x 5	
DAY 3: Cross-Training	
DAY 4: 3w/3r x 5	
DAY 5: Rest	
DAY 6: 3w/3r x 5	
DAY 7: Rest	

How did this week's runs go? Did I like them?
How did they make me feel?

What did I do for each cross-training workout?
Did I like it? How did it make me feel?

How much sleep did I get this week?
Was it enough?

How was my mental health this week?

Does anything hurt or feel sore on my body? If so, what have I done about it? (e.g., stretch, massage, etc.)

Anything else?

Week 7

What Was Scheduled	What You Actually Did
DAY 1: 2w/4r x 5	
DAY 2: Cross-Training	
DAY 3: 2w/4r x 5	
DAY 4: Cross-Training	
DAY 5: Rest	
DAY 6: 2w/4r x 5	
DAY 7: Rest	

How did this week's runs go? Did I like them?
How did they make me feel?

What did I do for each cross-training workout?
Did I like it? How did it make me feel?

How much sleep did I get this week?
Was it enough?

How was my mental health this week?

Does anything hurt or feel sore on my body? If so,
what have I done about it? (e.g., stretch, massage, etc.)

Anything else?

Week 8

What Was Scheduled	What You Actually Did
DAY 1: Cross-Training	
DAY 2: 2w/4r x 5	
DAY 3: Cross-Training	
DAY 4: 2w/4r x 5	
DAY 5: Rest	
DAY 6: 2w/4r x 5	
DAY 7: Rest	

How did this week's runs go? Did I like them?
How did they make me feel?

What did I do for each cross-training workout?
Did I like it? How did it make me feel?

How much sleep did I get this week?
Was it enough?

How was my mental health this week?

Does anything hurt or feel sore on my body? If so, what have I done about it? (e.g., stretch, massage, etc.)

Anything else?

Week 9

What Was Scheduled	What You Actually Did
DAY 1: 1w/5r x 5	
DAY 2: Cross-Training	
DAY 3: 1w/5r x 5	
DAY 4: Cross-Training	
DAY 5: Rest	
DAY 6: 1w/5r x 5	
DAY 7: Rest	

How did this week's runs go? Did I like them?
How did they make me feel?

What did I do for each cross-training workout?
Did I like it? How did it make me feel?

How much sleep did I get this week?
Was it enough?

How was my mental health this week?

Does anything hurt or feel sore on my body? If so, what have I done about it? (e.g., stretch, massage, etc.)

Anything else?

Week 10

What Was Scheduled	What You Actually Did
DAY 1: Cross-Training	
DAY 2: 1w/5r x 5	
DAY 3: Cross-Training	
DAY 4: 1w/5r x 5	
DAY 5: Rest	
DAY 6: 1w/5r x 5	
DAY 7: Rest	

How did this week's runs go? Did I like them?
How did they make me feel?

What did I do for each cross-training workout?
Did I like it? How did it make me feel?

How much sleep did I get this week?
Was it enough?

How was my mental health this week?

Does anything hurt or feel sore on my body? If so, what have I done about it? (e.g., stretch, massage, etc.)

Anything else?

Week 11

What Was Scheduled	What You Actually Did
DAY 1: Run 30 Minutes	
DAY 2: Cross-Training	
DAY 3: Run 30 Minutes	
DAY 4: Cross-Training	
DAY 5: Rest	
DAY 6: Run 30 Minutes	
DAY 7: Rest	

How did this week's runs go? Did I like them?
How did they make me feel?

What did I do for each cross-training workout?
Did I like it? How did it make me feel?

How much sleep did I get this week?
Was it enough?

How was my mental health this week?

Does anything hurt or feel sore on my body? If so,
what have I done about it? (e.g., stretch, massage, etc.)

Anything else?

Week 12

What Was Scheduled	What You Actually Did
DAY 1: Cross-Training	
DAY 2: Run 30 Minutes	
DAY 3: Cross-Training	
DAY 4: Run 3 Miles* *Yes, this one is different! It lets you see what it feels like to run by miles, not minutes.*	
DAY 5: Rest	
DAY 6: Run 30 Minutes	
DAY 7: Rest	

How did this week's runs go? Did I like them?
How did they make me feel?

What did I do for each cross-training workout?
Did I like it? How did it make me feel?

How did it feel to run 3 miles on Day 4?
Do I prefer running by mileage or time?

How much sleep did I get this week?
Was it enough?

How was my mental health this week?

Does anything hurt or feel sore on my body? If so, what have I done about it? (e.g., stretch, massage, etc.)

Reflections
After You Finish the Three
Month Training Program

What was my "why" for each day's cross-training or run?

What was the best part of these three months?

If I was nervous anything before starting this program, were my fears justified? Did other fears come up during the three months? Do I still have them?

What did I learn from these three months? Was the experience different from what I expected?

What's Next?

You finished!!! That is amazing and fantastic. I am impressed, and you should be too. So, what's next on your running journey? Not sure yet? Take some time to fill out the optional end-of-program reflection pages.

If you want to keep running, just keep it up! You're doing great. Know that it is *much easier* to just keep running than to start again. And now that you've finished this program, you have lots of options. Try these:

Prefer the cadence of run/walk over just running?
Repeat Weeks 5 and 6 of the training plan for as long as you want.

Want to keep running but not increase how much time you spend running each week?

Keep repeating Week 11 of the training program. Running thirty minutes three times a week (plus two cross-training workouts) is wonderful. If you don't want to do more than that, don't.

You'd like to keep increasing how much you're running?

Great. Slowly and safely increase how much you run—both in terms of number of runs each week and the length of those runs. You can do this by following existing training plans—Hal Higdon (HalHigdon.com), Runner's World Magazine (RunnersWorld.com), and Trail Runner Magazine (TrailRunnerMag.com) all have great ones. Pick an "easy" plan that starts off at about nine total miles (or less) per week.

Want personalized help to get after some big running goals?

Hire a coach to give you a personalized training plan. You can find great coaches through Road Runners Club of America (Rrca.org/Coaches) or North Coast Running (NorthCoastRunning.com). Coaches usually work with you remotely, so it doesn't really matter where you and they live. I've worked with coaches at North Coast Running for a few years now and really love it.

There's a whole community of runners out there. I promise they're all excited you've joined them in this silly but wonderful thing called running. You'll find them on runs, at shoe stores, local races, and just about everywhere else. Joining a local running club is a great way to make more friends and find people with a wealth of knowledge about running.

Congrats on becoming a runner!

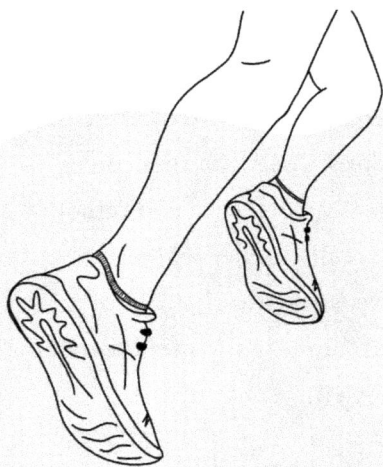

About the Author

Sarah Austin Casson is a runner and environmental anthropologist who has helped countless others to become runners. She firmly believes the point of running is to have fun.

Running lets Casson wander new places and discover familiar ones. It has brought her new friends and deepened relationships with old ones.

Casson has run (and worked) all over the world. She has worked with farmers, wilderness rangers, policymakers, scientists, and others to look at some of our gnarliest problems: climate change, collapsed prehistoric societies, wilderness conservation, and more. She's interested in how we interact with one another and the natural environment, how we conceptualize our worlds, and what it means to exist in the nuances our world demands.

You'll find her eating delicious food in dense cities and goofing around in remote wildernesses. She's climbed volcanoes, summited mountains, dived deep into the oceans, and traversed jungles. Wherever she travels, her running shoes always come along.

She can be found online at:

SarahAustinCasson.com